Mind The Gut

How To Heal Your Gut From The Inside Out

Sarah Spann

Mind The Gut © Copyright 2020 Sarah Spann

ISBN: 978-0-6489355-0-6

First published 2020

All rights reserved. No part of this publication may be reproduced, distributed or transmitted in any form or by any means, including photocopying, recording, or other electronic or mechanical methods, without the prior written permission of the author, except in the case of brief quotations embodied in critical reviews and certain other noncommercial uses permitted by copyright law.

Neither the author nor the publisher can be held responsible for the use of the information provided within this book. Please always consult a trained professional before making any decision regarding treatment of yourself or others.

Email sarah@sarahspann.net

Web sarahspann.net

Dedication

For my husband, Matthew, and all my family, friends, mentors and supporters without whom this book would never have happened.

Thank you for your wisdom, advice and encouragement.

Table of Contents

Prelude 1

Chapter 1 – A Gut Wrenching System 3

Chapter 2 – The Gut Garden 13

Chapter 3 – Gut Central 21

Chapter 4 – The Holistic Element 27

Chapter 5 – The Gut Soothing Blueprint 35

Chapter 6 – Determining Your Diet 41

Chapter 7 – Your Gut is You 47

Chapter 8 – Taming Tension 53

Chapter 9 – Supercharge Your Self Love 61

Chapter 10 – Sustainable Solutions 71

Chapter 11 – Harmonious Healing 79

Chapter 12 – Infusing Inspiration 87

References 97

About The Author 99

Prelude

Do you feel like you're stuck in a never-ending cycle of gut issues?

Are you constantly feeling frustrated because your symptoms are dictating where you can go, what you can wear, what you can do and who you can see?

Are you anxious about eating because you seem to react to every food every single time?

Do you feel like you are trying so hard to get better and yet nothing seems to last long-term?

If you answered yes to any of these questions, this book will show you how to:

- Relieve your gut symptoms quickly
- Get your diet right for your body
- Find out what has been keeping you stuck
- Easily manage your symptoms and live a normal life without the stress of constant gut flare-ups

Even if you thought it was impossible.

Even if nothing ever seems to work.

Even if you've been dealing with your symptoms for decades.

In this book you'll discover:

- Why you are not doomed to live with unrelenting gut issues forever

- Why nothing has worked yet and what to do instead

- A holistic approach that addresses all factors that cause you to suffer from gut issues

- How to come back to the you that existed before all this happened

Chapter 1 – A Gut Wrenching System

"Free yourself from the inauthenticity and disempowerment of your story" – Steve Maraboli

When it comes to the gut, many people fall into a disempowering system.

If you're reading this book, I'm sure you've felt the frustrations that come along with gut issues that seem to get worse no matter what you do or try.

Why is it that when you have a digestive issue, it's so difficult to find answers? Why is it that something will work for someone else, and not for you? Why is it that you're always the person that can't be explained? And where do you go from here?

The more interest that grows in gut health, the more confusing it will get. There will only be more opinions, more cure-all diets, more supplements and more conflicting evidence.

Before I go any further, let me share with you why I'm writing this book.

When I was in my teenage years, I started to become quite unwell. I was always bloated, I had headaches and felt tired and sick all the time. When I was younger, I didn't pay too much attention to it, but as the years went on, I got more and more unwell and my stomach was a mess.

When I was about 19, I ended up being hospitalized because of severe stomach cramps. After being given some heavy painkillers and doing a bunch of tests, I was told it was a UTI that was causing this severe pain. During the next week, I went to more doctors, had more tests, but no one knew what was going on. I spent that week knocked out on pain killers.

Things continued to get worse. I was exhausted, hiding, and being anti-social because I was too tired to do anything. I was too tired to exercise, and I was always going home from work because I was feeling sick in the stomach. I worked in corporate from age 19 and it was very distressing having to go home sick in an environment that expects so much.

Interestingly, my younger sister was going through stomach concerns at the same time. She was trying different diets and having different tests done, which prompted me to look at my diet too. I started eating healthier and tried cutting out different foods, but nothing seemed to help. Eventually, one GP suggested screening for coeliac disease. I was about 23 by this point.

After the screening tests came back positive, I had an endoscopy and colonoscopy which confirmed that I did have coeliac disease.

Coeliac disease is an autoimmune reaction to the protein gluten which is found in wheat, barley malt and rye. The protein in oats is avenin which not all coeliacs react to, but oats are often cross-contaminated with gluten-containing crops.

Essentially what happens in coeliac disease is, this protein causes an autoimmune reaction in the body resulting in extensive damage in the small intestine.

The small intestine is the absorption centre of the body and is where 90% of absorption happens. If the small intestine was all laid out, it would be almost the surface area of a football field. The small intestine is lined with finger-like projections called villi. In coeliac disease, the body attacks the villi and they become flat and inflamed. It's like a chainsaw has been taken to them and chopped them off.

This means that you don't absorb anything from food. So not only do you end up with malnutrition but if left untreated, you can end up with cardiovascular problems, secondary autoimmune conditions, depression, anxiety, osteoporosis and even lymphoma (similar to any untreated gut problem).

The good news was, it explained why I was so unwell and why I had been losing weight. It was good to finally get some answers. When I had my scopes done, I remember the gastroenterologist telling me that my villi were 'flat as a tack' and that I needed to stop eating gluten so that I don't die. Knowing what I do now, I don't think he was being dramatic.

Transitioning to gluten free had its own challenges. It wasn't as common knowledge then as it is now. The knowledge on coeliac disease was still emerging and it was more difficult to find gluten free food. Gluten free bread has also come a long way!

After about four months on a gluten free diet, I felt like a new person. I had energy again, I could exercise, go to work, *and* socialize in the same day, which was huge for me considering I used to struggle just to complete a full day of work. I was in such a better mood; I was putting on weight and I felt happy.

However, even though I was much better, I still had IBS symptoms going on, and things did get to a point where they plateaued. They even started going backwards, and a whole bunch of other physical and emotional problems started happening. Then I fell back into the system of 'we don't know what's wrong'.

I had been wanting to start studying nutritional medicine for quite some time, but I was torn because I also wanted to spend a few years living in the UK. In an interesting twist of fate, I met my (now) husband just as I was about to leave on this trip. A couple of years turned into 4 months, and I started studying when I returned home.

I wanted to study for me because I hadn't been able to find any answers, but I also wanted to understand how food works in the body specifically so that I could help other people to eat right for their body and feed themselves the foods that their body loves and needs too.

One thing that studying helped me with, was understanding what was happening inside my body. Whilst it was explained to me that I needed to stop eating gluten, it wasn't explained that due to the extent of the damage, some serious gut repair work was required.

The other big discovery I made was the influence of emotions on the gut, and my emotional healing journey became integral to my gut recovery as well.

Many of my clients felt like they had to turn themselves into a study case as well. A gut health journey (or any health journey really) is often a world of confusion and frustration. It can be a real trial and error type situation which can feel like two steps forwards and three back.

Clients have shared with me that they usually get told something along the lines of 'it's probably IBS, take these pills, try the low FODMAP diet and stress less' (FODMAP is an acronym for fermentable oligosaccharides, disaccharides, monosaccharides and polyols – a group of short-chain carbohydrate foods that are commonly poorly absorbed).

But IBS is a disempowering diagnosis because it literally shuts down the process of investigating what's causing it. The thing is, your gut symptoms aren't happening because of IBS. Something is happening in your body and IBS is the diagnosis you have been given.

But this isn't how IBS is viewed in the mainstream. You often get put on standard protocols that don't work, your diet becomes more restricted, and your symptoms get worse because no investigation is being done into what's really causing them.

Unfortunately, people often get stuck on restrictive diets long-term, such as a low FODMAP diet, because whenever they try to reintroduce foods their symptoms return. This happens when the core gut healing work hasn't been done.

Elimination of restrictive diets are intended to be transitional. Diets of this nature cut out many beneficial fibres that the gut needs and can create nutritional deficiencies and more gut problems when used long-term.

Not to mention the emotional and psychological stress that comes with living on an extremely restricted diet.

In the current system, there's also no consideration of the long-term consequences of relying on pills and medications, which is especially important given the impact that these medications have on the gut microbiome (discussed later in this book).

You're told to 'stress less' without any discussion on what stress really is, how it impacts your body, how the whole system is connected or how you, in fact, 'stress less' when you're walking out with the same pressures and demands that were on you when you went in. Not to mention that your digestive issues are probably the biggest source of your stress!

We desperately need a new approach to gut health. An approach that is holistic and empowering. An approach that helps you to understand what your symptoms mean. An approach that teaches you how to listen to your body. An approach that focuses on total body wellness where the physical, emotional, and energetic bodies are all included.

The new approach needs to consider what our lives are and how we can approach gut healing from a different angle. It needs to ensure that all factors causing the gut issues are addressed, but in a way, that's practical, doable and sustainable.

The body is a self-healing organism and it has an innate ability to heal, given the right circumstances. It's a matter of discovering what's right for you and giving your body what it needs.

Modern medicine is amazing. It saves millions of lives and has kept generations of humans alive. But one big difference between the two is that modern medicine shines when you can physically see the problem, and naturopathic medicine shines when you can't. Naturopathic nutritionists, such as I, are trained to look at the whole body, rather than individual pieces. Naturopathic medicine has been treating the gut for centuries.

You need to feel empowered when it comes to your body. When you understand what's going on in your body, when you know what the signals mean, and when you know how to give your body what it needs to heal and why it enables true healing. I do believe that everyone can heal with the right guidance and direction.

Too many people are suffering and it's time to take the power back instead of getting swallowed up in a disempowered system. It's also important to never give up. You don't have to accept that things will always be this way, that your condition is who you are and that nothing can be done. There is *always* something that can be done to improve your health and your quality of life.

This book is going to show you a unique approach to gut health that you haven't been told about before. It delivers a holistic solution that addresses all factors that cause you to suffer from gut issues. It shows you how to care for your gut and delivers the things which will help every single person, no matter what your circumstances are or whatever other treatments you are having.

Once I discovered this approach, and I came out the other side, life has been so different. I can now focus and concentrate on things without falling asleep. I can sleep through the night instead of being up all night with reflux or a racing mind.

I don't stress about toilet locations and I don't have the stress of knowing that I will probably have to use public toilets any time I go out. I don't get anxious about bloating or gas.

I know how to listen to my body and I immediately know if I've eaten something that didn't suit me – and I know straight away what it was. My gut doesn't flare up whenever I get stressed anymore.

I still need to ask questions and be vigilant when eating out, but it doesn't bother me because I now know what questions to ask. Also, any flare-ups I do get from food these days are minor, and I recover quickly.

With any gut-related disorder, there will always be maintenance things to do. The difference is knowing what those things are as opposed to guessing in the dark. Because once you know exactly how to manage your gut, your life totally changes.

And all of this is possible for you too, no matter how hard it's been hard so far.

I used to be scared to leave the house and now here I am writing a book!

The truth is that the way to heal your gut is to heal your life.

Chapter 2 – The Gut Garden

"We do not inherit the microbiota from our ancestors, we borrow it from our children" – Jason Hawrelak

Digestive disorders are on the rise. You only need to look at all the marketing and fascination with gut health to see how the world is focusing on the gut.

As we should be.

25% (1 in 4) people in Australia, and the USA, have irritable bowel syndrome (IBS)[2]. 11% of the global population have IBS[1]. Further, in 2017 there were 6.8 million cases of IBD globally, which is a substantial increase from cases of IBD since 1990[3].

Inflammatory bowel disease (IBD) is also becoming more prevalent, more complex, and more severe. In 2013, 75,000 (1 in 250) people in Australia had IBD and this number was projected to increase to 100,000 by 2022[4]. As of 2017, 1.6 million Americans had Crohn's Disease or Ulcerative Colitis. And there are 70,000 new cases each year[5].

Obviously, this has huge consequences, not only on quality of life but also economic consequences for both those affected and our health system.

Aside from the impact that gut issues have on your life in the short term (like fatigue, unpredictable stomach upsets, bloating, pain, embarrassing symptoms, missing out on things and fears of eating out), there are also long-term consequences to unaddressed gut symptoms such as depression, anxiety, obesity, and autoimmune disease.

But before we embark on this journey of gut healing, it's important to understand what the gut is, its role in the body and how things go wrong.

[Note: this is intended to be a general overview of the gut, not an extensive explanation. For more detail I suggest reading *Gut: The Inside Story of The Body's Most Underrated Organ* by Giulia Enders].

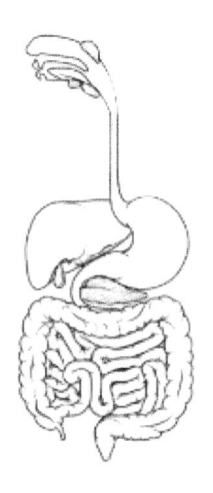

Source: Canva

There are trillions of bacteria in the gut, containing over 500 species and weighing around 1.3kg. The bacterial DNA outnumber your own DNA by over 100 times. You have about 23,000 genes, but there are 3.3 million or more bacterial genes (this figure is in debate and will probably change as we learn more, but either way, we are literally more bacteria than human).

Think of it like this – we don't tolerate the gut bugs, they tolerate us!

Some of the many things the gut microbiome does for us include:

- Strengthening the immune system and protection against allergy development

- Maintaining gut motility to ensure that food passes through properly

- Nutrient absorption and metabolism

- Maintenance of the lining of the intestinal tract

- Influence on weight management through their role in energy balance

- Influence on blood sugar control

- Regulation of mood

Your gut exists as a delicate ecosystem. It's like a garden with flowers, trees, plants, soil, grass, weeds and all the creatures that live there.

A healthy garden will have few weeds, many plants and flowers, perhaps some trees, herbs, vegetables and healthy soil. It will be tended to regularly – fertilised, watered and loved. In a neglected garden, weeds have overtaken the plants. Flowers are dying, creatures are leaving, the soil is barren and dry.

When we have a healthy garden, all systems work well and support each other. But when the balance is thrown out, we go into chaos.

The three major gut disruptors are diet, stress, and the environment.

The typical Western diet is not beneficial for our gut. The beneficial bacteria need plenty of fibre to survive, and because there are so many species of bacteria in the gut, they need many kinds of fibres from a wide variety of fruits and vegetables. This is where the saying 'eat a rainbow' becomes especially important.

Our gut bacteria are involved in everything that happens to our body, and they live off fibre. They need a wide variety of fibre to thrive and populate a healthy colony.

Only 42% of children and 28% of adults in Australia meet the Australian Government recommendations for fibre intake. On top of this, 92% of Australian adults do not eat the daily recommended vegetable intake.

In conjunction with this, our consumption of 'discretionary foods' – processed foods, sugary drinks, cakes, biscuits, chips, deep-fried foods etc – is increasing in Australian children, accounting for 41% of the energy intake, or 6-8 serves, in children aged 14-18. These foods are energy dense and nutrient poor, meaning that they are empty calories with no nutritional value.

We know that these foods disrupt the gut microbiome and create inflammation in the gut.

One issue is that we are hardwired to crave sugar, fat, and salt because historically, these foods gave us energy in times of famine. We are no longer in famine, but our DNA doesn't know that yet. And the food industry is *very* aware of this. Food companies spend thousands, if not more, on research to find that perfect combination of sugar, fat, and salt to keep you coming back for more.

Stress is also a great disruptor of the microbiome. Ever felt that 'kick in the guts' sensation, butterflies or the feeling of a sinking stomach? The need to run to the bathroom when you're nervous? These are all examples of the microbes reacting to stress.

Research into this area is showing us that depressed people have higher levels of inflammatory bacteria and lower levels of beneficial bacteria in the gut.

The pressures and demands of life are increasing. We're being asked to work more and do more with less. We've got financial pressures, work pressures and family pressures. This drives an inflammatory response in the body which affects the gut, and I'll explain this connection in much more detail in the next chapter.

We've got more toxins in our environment than ever before in history. Chemicals and endocrine disruptors in our personal care products, cleaning products, plastics, fumes and pesticides. This use of chemicals is impacting not only our gut microbiome, but newer research suggests that it's also impacting the gut microbiome of animals exposed to these toxins, including bees.

We know that antibiotics, proton pump inhibitors and non-steroidal anti-inflammatories negatively impact the balance of bacteria in the gut, and these medications are used extensively.

These factors make up the disappearing microbiome theory. The theory is that as generations go on, the diversity and the number of species of bacteria in our guts is decreasing.

One study compared the microbiome of people in the Hadza tribe of Tanzania against the microbiome of Westerners. The diversity score was found to be 5 times higher in the Hadza tribe, which is thought to be because of their high-quality fibre diet, differences in lifestyle and lower toxin exposure[6].

What this means is that certain gut bacteria that carry out specific roles in the body are dying off, and they're not returning. Which is affecting not only our health but the health of future generations. What happens with our gut microbiome can impact our entire lineage.

It's critical that we get a handle on this because if we don't, the rates of digestive issues are going to continue to increase. Children will get sicker at younger ages, and adults will suffer higher rates of chronic disease.

But the world isn't going to change anytime soon. Sure, there is a push towards more healthy and sustainable ways of living, but in conjunction with this, there's also a push to keep things the way they are. It's not that simple to change a world of convenience eating, fast paced living and chemical use.

So, it's really important to take care of your gut garden. Love it, tend to it, nurture it and look after it.

Key Take-Aways

- Diversity in the gut microbiota (having many different species of bacteria living in the gut) is essential because they all have different roles in the body

- Choose fresh, whole foods over processed, sugary junk

- Be mindful of your stress and your environment

- Treat your gut the way you would treat a garden that you love. Feed it, water it, nurture it and don't poison it

Chapter 3 – Gut Central

"Quite literally, your gut is the epicentre of your physical and mental health. If you want better immunity, efficient digestion, improved clarity and balance, focus on rebuilding your gut health" – Kris Carr.

Problems in the gut do not just stay in the gut.

This is because of the central role the gut plays in all aspects of health. Anything that happens in the gut has a ripple effect throughout the entire body. This is why you'll also be getting concomitant problems like fatigue, brain fog, irritability, anxiety, hormonal disruptions and difficulty sleeping.

The positive side of this, however, is that the ripple effect goes both ways.

When I work with clients, they report back to me that as their gut symptoms disappear, they also feel mentally clearer, more energetic, more confident, relieved, sleep better, are able to exercise more and feel much better in themselves. Many of my clients even lose weight as an added bonus.

One of my clients, we'll call her Melanie, had been experiencing itchy rashes down the sides of her legs, purple marks on her feet and terrible headaches. Once we did some gut healing work and got her diet right specifically for her,

her headaches subsided, and her rashes and purple marks disappeared. This all happened within a matter of weeks.

The way that problems in the gut end up outside of the gut happens in 3 stages.

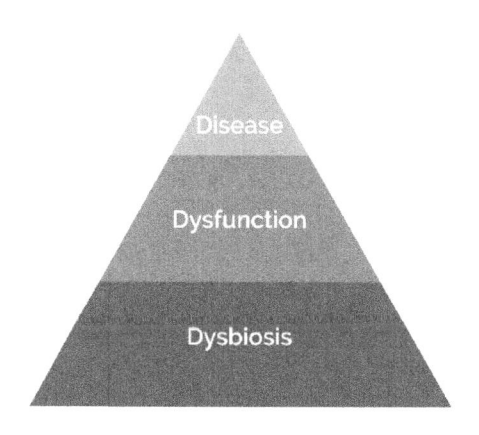

Pyramid diagram with three tiers from top to bottom: Disease, Dysfunction, Dysbiosis.

Dysbiosis

Dysbiosis means that there has been a change in the gut bacteria that is causing harmful effects. The previous chapters discussed how this happens.

Using our garden analogy, in the gut, we have lovely plants like *Lactobacillus* and *Bifidobacteria*, and weeds like pathogens and parasites. They both belong there, but the amount of each type should be in balance.

Bacterial infections can kill you, so it's no surprise that the body runs into trouble when the balance of bacteria in the gut is out of whack.

Dysfunction

The gut is lined with a complex intestinal barrier. This is what keeps the gut bacteria and food particles inside the gut, where they should stay.

An unhealthy gut garden compromises this barrier. Certain flowers are kept in greenhouses to protect them from external elements. Imagine if the greenhouse was taken away and they had to fend for themselves.

When the intestinal barrier is compromised, it is called intestinal permeability or more commonly, leaky gut.

The bacteria that leak out of the gut and into the bloodstream induce systemic inflammation in the body and damage body tissues and organs. It also hyper-stimulates the immune system because your immune system launches an attack on the bacteria. Many immune compounds are also synthesised in the gut.

This situation is a bit like the cane toad problem in Australia. Cane toads are useful in their natural habitat, but when they were brought to Australia, they attacked all the native animals, disrupted the ecosystem, and have changed the face of the environment forever.

Disease

At this point the immune system is overstimulated, there is body-wide inflammation and other organs are being affected. Body systems can't operate efficiently.

It's like a fire raging inside your body. Unless we put it out, it will continue to damage the body and creates further problems outside of the gut like depression, anxiety, obesity, insulin resistance, migraines, skin rashes or autoimmune disease.

But this process isn't the only way that the gut bacteria impact your entire body and brain.

Let's revisit the gut garden analogy. In a healthy garden the flowers would provide pollen for the bees, the worms would regenerate the soil, and the roots of the trees would go deep into the Earth to support new growth. It all functions together in a perfect ecosystem.

In the gut, the many different bacteria play different roles in the body. This is why it's so important that we have as many different species in there as possible. Imagine if all the flowers disappeared from a garden – where would the bees go?

Certain microbiota produce neurotransmitters including serotonin and dopamine. In fact, the majority of production of these neurotransmitters takes place in the gut. Serotonin is associated with happiness or contentment, and dopamine with reward or pleasure.

If there is an overgrowth of weeds (like lipopolysaccharides or candida) in place of the neurotransmitter producing flowers, it can create imbalanced neurotransmitter status in the body which is a biochemical cause of depression.

It's so important that we maintain the health of our gut garden. That we love it, tend to it, fertilise it and care for it. And one simple way that you can look after your gut garden is to nourish it with prebiotic and probiotic foods.

Prebiotics are like fertiliser. They provide food for the flowers and plants in your gut garden to ensure that they can grow and the environment is set up to thrive. Whereas taking probiotics is like planting flowers in your garden directly. However, if the soil isn't watered and fertilised, these flowers will die. This is one reason to have both prebiotics and probiotics in your diet.

You'll get plenty of prebiotics through eating lovely fibrous foods – fruit, vegetables, nuts, seeds, whole grains and legumes. Fermented foods like sauerkraut, kim chi and yogurt are great sources of probiotics.

Supplementation can also be very helpful given that our gut garden is up against a lot of toxic agents in our diet, lifestyles and environment. However, the supplement industry is huge and confusing. It's best to get professional advice before going out and spending hundreds on products that may not work or even make you feel worse.

Key Take-Aways

- What happens in the gut doesn't stay in the gut, but you can solve many problems by correcting the gut

- The gut bacteria belong in the gut. When the intestinal barrier is compromised the bacteria leak out into the bloodstream, attacking joints and DNA

- The resulting immune system response creates further disruption and disease in the body

- Prebiotics are fertiliser for your gut garden and are found in fibrous foods

- Probiotics are like directly planting the flowers in the garden and are in fermented foods

Chapter 4 – The Holistic Element

"The body is a self-healing organism, so it's really about clearing things out of the way so the body can heal itself" – Barbara Brennan

We aren't a society that typically accepts pain.

Many of us have been conditioned to 'pop a pill and get on with it', to never speak of pain, ignore it and keep going. Be tough. There's no time to be feeling sorry for yourself!

Not long after my diagnosis of coeliac disease, I decided I wanted to run a half marathon. I started training with a friend of mine who was a former triathlete. During one of our first 10km runs, I sprained my ankle about 4km in. I didn't stop running. Yes, my ankle was hurting, but I was so determined to finish the 10km.

The result was that I created a huge mess of my ankle, and I couldn't run at all for weeks. I needed crutches and physiotherapy to recover. I couldn't do the half marathon, but I did at least manage to do the 10km leg.

We have pain mechanisms in the body for a reason. The pain is a warning sign. When you put your hand on a hot surface, the pain mechanism warns you to move away so that you don't burn. If the pain mechanism wasn't there, your hand could burn off and you would have no idea.

The pain in your gut might be annoying right now, but it might also be a sign of underlying disease. The pain won't go away. It will just get louder until you're forced to attend to it.

If you've had the physical checks done and there was nothing physically wrong, you may have been diagnosed with irritable bowel syndrome (IBS).

IBS essentially means that you're getting gut symptoms like unpredictable bowel movements, reflux, nausea, constipation and diarrhoea without any visible signs of damage or disease in your digestive system. It can leave you feeling like your gut is playing up for no apparent reason.

Except there's always a reason. If your system is not operating the way it should be, there *is* a reason and there is always something we can do about it. There's never a situation where it can't be improved. It doesn't matter how long you've had this problem, or how long you've been suffering, or what you've been told.

There's always something we can do when a holistic approach is taken. It's simply a matter of digging deeper and peeling back the layers on what's happening biochemically, physically, emotionally, environmentally and energetically and addressing that to allow the body to heal.

When you have a gut condition, things will never be 'perfect'. There will be maintenance things you need to do, foods that you'll need to avoid and cautions that you'll need to take. But knowing what these things are is where the empowerment comes from.

There's so much we can do from a natural perspective. There are so many techniques and remedies that soothe the gut, settle digestion and improve your symptoms before even looking at diet (although diet is very important too!). These are things that you can do yourself, and things that you'll need to do in order to heal the gut, no matter what other treatments you are having. You'll learn more about this in later chapters.

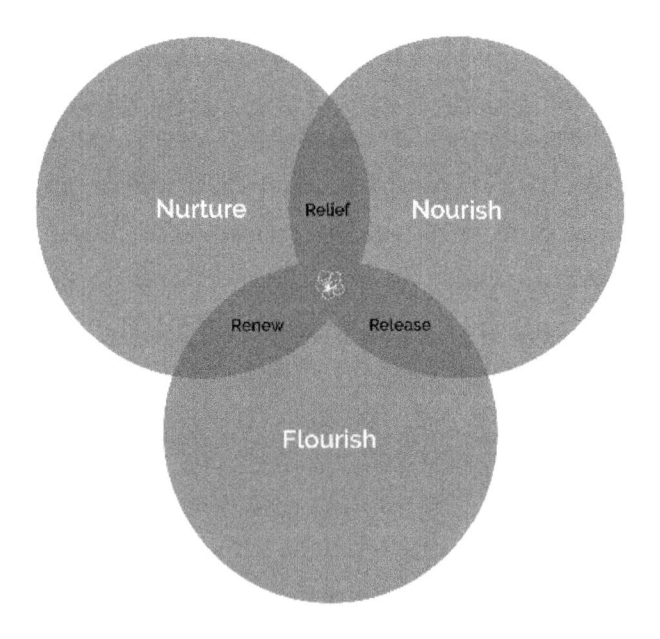

[Venn diagram with three overlapping circles labeled Nurture, Nourish, and Flourish. The overlapping regions are labeled Relief (Nurture ∩ Nourish), Renew (Nurture ∩ Flourish), and Release (Nourish ∩ Flourish).]

To heal your gut, it's so important to identify how to nurture your body with what it needs to heal, and this is what will be covered in this book.

Once you know how to nurture your body and you understand the signals you're getting, you need to be ok with acting on those messages. This is where nourish comes in.

We sometimes hear that little voice telling us to slow down, to say no to something, not eat something, stop eating now, or do gentle exercise over intense today. But 90% of the time we'll be too busy, too stressed or feeling like it's unacceptable to take a break because there's so much going on, we're needed in 20 different directions and we'll sleep when we're dead.

One of my clients, let's call her Tracey, experienced this first-hand. She was getting constant wind and stomach pain; she was exhausted, and she felt nauseous constantly. After we began our work together, she had started to recover from these symptoms and was doing really well.

However, suddenly, in the space of literally one week, she went downhill. She put on weight, she felt exhausted, she was anxious, and all her gut symptoms were coming back. But nothing had changed in her diet, or in her life.

When we dove a little deeper into this, we uncovered that she had been doing far too much for other people, worrying about what others were thinking of her and working herself into the ground to keep everyone else happy. This was driving a massive stress response in the body. After we did some work around this, she's been on the up and up ever since.

The impact of stress on the gut is huge because the body has a physiological response to stress. When the body perceives danger, it activates what is called the 'sympathetic nervous system' (SNS), or the 'flight or fight' response.

The stress response is ancient. The body does not know what the thought is – just how it makes it feel. Your body still believes that when you feel stressed, anxious, depressed or flustered that you are in physical danger and prepares you accordingly. It's just trying to keep you alive. The world has evolved far too quickly for our bodies to keep up.

The SNS tells the body to secrete the stress hormones cortisol and adrenaline. It also draws blood away from your digestive tract and to your arms and legs to prepare you to run or fight, because your body believes your life is in danger. There is no need to digest your food right now. In fact, your body will try and get *rid* of food to make it lighter. As a result, your digestion becomes impaired and food doesn't get absorbed properly.

If you constantly have adrenaline and cortisol pumping through your blood because of the thought patterns running through your head and the pressures that you feel, and because of this you never allow yourself to rest, the world's best diet and supplements won't be enough. You may feel better in the short-term, but it won't last. Your mental and emotional health is just as much a part of the picture as your physical health.

So, it's pretty simple, eat healthy and stress less, right?

I don't know about you, but I find it infuriating when someone tells me to 'chill out' when I'm stressed to the max. Also, the reality is that we all *know* we need to eat healthy and stress less. Simply being told this isn't helpful.

This is why we need a holistic approach, which is being delivered in this book. When you have this foundation, you can become truly well from the inside out and live life on your terms, rather than based on what's happening with your gut that day.

Whether you'd like to have enough energy to work, exercise and socialise in the same day (which used to be impossible for me), go on a long-haul flight without having to get up 20 times for the toilet, or go to lunch without any anxiety – this is absolutely possible for you. I've seen it time, and time, and time again.

This is the work that will end the control of your gut and your symptoms on your life. When you do this work, you have the insight and intuition to give your body what it loves and needs. You have the courage and confidence to do the right thing by you, and you get back the motivation to go out there and flourish.

Key Take-Aways

- Being diagnosed with a digestive disorder doesn't mean there's nothing more that can be done

- Using a holistic approach that encourages you to nurture your body rather than trying to force symptoms to go away is far more effective and empowering

- The physiological stress response activates the sympathetic nervous system (SNS) which essentially shuts down digestion and creates gut symptoms

- Listen to that little voice steering you away from stressful foods and situations

Chapter 5 – The Gut Soothing Blueprint

"Every moment nature is serving fresh dishes with the items of happiness. It is our choice to recognize and taste it" – Amit Ray

Now that you understand the role of the gut and what a gut garden does, the next step is to optimise your digestion and settle your gut symptoms.

The way you eat your food matters even more so than what the food is. Have you ever been told to slow down, chew your food, sit down for a meal? Well, there's a very good reason for that.

When I eat constantly standing up and on the run, when I shovel my food in because I've got too much else to do, essentially ignoring my own advice by eating and working at the same time without focusing on the food, my bloating certainly is a lot worse. And I'm crankier.

Many of my clients find that they have less bloating, cramping and gas simply by eating their meals away from the TV, books, phones or laptops.

The digestive system is like a factory production line. It's very systematic. One thing needs to happen at one step before it can happen at the next step. If the machine breaks at one point, it affects the next and so on.

This entire factory is controlled by the vagus nerve, which is the longest nerve in the body and is connected to several parts of the gut. The vagus nerve is also like the switch that flicks on the digestive system. It prompts the body to start secreting digestive juices and it initiates contractions in the digestive tract which moves the food through the system.

Before eating, we need to activate the vagus nerve. The good news is that there is a fun way to do this – the vagus nerve responds to happiness!

So, you could smile, laugh, sing, or do a quick dance around the kitchen – or simply take 3-5 deep belly breaths and think about the meal that's on the way. This will flick the switch and start your digestion factory.

Once the factory is on, we need to make sure that it operates efficiently. Digestion starts in the mouth, with saliva and chewing. You start salivating before a meal to help digest carbohydrates. If you don't chew your food properly, your stomach has a very difficult task ahead of it, especially if you also haven't activated the vagus nerve and switched on the system itself.

The small intestine is the absorption centre of the body, where 90% of absorption happens. The pancreas secrete digestive enzymes, and the liver makes bile which is stored in the gallbladder and secreted into the small intestines to help this process. However, these mechanisms are only activated once they receive a signal from the stomach, and the vagus nerve.

If food hasn't been broken down properly by the stomach, it won't be broken down and absorbed properly by the small intestines because the food particles are too large to go through the walls of the small intestine. It means that this food ends up fermenting in the colon instead, creating pain, gas, constipation, diarrhoea, nausea and bloating. It also drives inflammatory responses by the immune system which causes you to become sensitive to more and more foods. This is a big reason it can feel like the list of foods you can eat keeps shrinking.

The bottom line is that it's not what you eat, it's what you absorb. If you're constantly eating on the run, shovelling food in whilst distracted and working, all the while your mind is going one million miles an hour – you're not getting anything from your food and even worse, it's upsetting your gut.

It's so important to activate your vagus nerve and eat properly so that your digestive system is working optimally. Think of food as a source of nourishment, enjoyment, and medicine. Be grateful for the meal, for this fuel that is keeping you alive. This alone is going to change your gut symptoms significantly.

The main message here is, eat kindly for your body and give your body the best chance. These methods sound simple, but I promise you, this alone is going to allow your body to start to heal and help to decrease your symptoms, allowing you more freedom with food.

I know that it can be very difficult to eat in this way with our fast-paced lifestyles, and it may not always be possible. But if you can make a conscious effort to try and do it as much as you can, it's really going to make such a difference.

As for what to eat, the short answer is to go for a predominantly fresh, whole foods diet with plenty of vegetables, some fruit, nuts, seeds, lean protein and healthy fats. The long answer is in the next chapter.

Remember too that chemicals also disrupt the gut. Buy organic produce where possible and if you can't, wash non-organic produce in apple cider vinegar before consuming it. Choose natural personal care and cleaning products – your skin is an absorption organ too! Help your gut garden thrive.

A note on intermittent fasting

I wanted to touch on intermittent fasting because it's another popular topic that is slightly controversial. Certainly, it does have benefits for the gut with some studies showing that intermittent fasting improves gut barrier integrity and restores normal microflora. However, it's important to get professional advice with your situation, as fasting doesn't work for everyone.

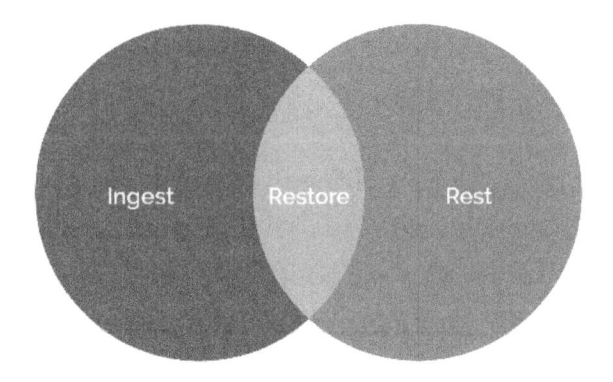

Ingest — Restore — Rest

After ingestion of food, you need to have a period of rest to allow the digestive system to restore. About 3 hours after a meal, a mechanism called the Migrating Motor Complex (MMC) is activated. This is like a cleaner coming through an office and cleaning up all the trash from the day. However, if you continually eat, this complex doesn't get activated and the digestive 'rubbish' continues to pile up.

So, it's important to take breaks between meals as constant grazing is not helpful for your digestion. However, if you want to look at fasting, make sure you plan properly and get some professional advice. Personally, I allow 12-14 hours between dinner and breakfast. I find this helps my system to reset.

Activity

Choose at least two actions from the list below and implement them every day this week. Notice how your gut feels.

- Squeeze ½ fresh lemon in a large glass of warm water and drink each morning

- Avoid water with meals and add fresh lemon juice or 1 tsp apple cider vinegar if drinking liquids with a meal

- Add bitter foods – rocket, olives, lemon juice – to meals

- Drink dandelion tea before or after meals

- Eat gut friendly, easily digestible foods such as broths, soups, stews, and slow cooked meals

- Eat meals away from distractions

- Take 3-5 deep breaths before starting your meal (or smile and laugh!)

- Chew 20-30 times per mouthful

Chapter 6 – Determining Your Diet

"The food you eat can be either the safest and most powerful form of medicine or the slowest form of poison" – Ann Wigmore

Whenever people find out what I do, the first question is often 'what should I eat?'

While I was studying and learning all about food, eating became very stressful for me. Every time I would eat something, I'd think about all the negatives of that food (there are negatives to all foods, even blueberries!). I'd think about where the food came from, how it had been prepared and whether, as a nutritionist, I should be eating it. I was very conscious of what I ate in front of others and felt the pressure to eat 'perfectly' (that doesn't exist by the way).

So, what should you eat? Should you go gluten free, vegan, paleo, pescatarian, flexitarian, carnivore, Atkins, fasting… what's right?

All the conflicting information and new viewpoints coming out on diet every single day can make things very overwhelming.

The truth is that diet is very individual and it's going to be different for everyone. There are going to be foods that upset you, and not someone else. There are going to be foods that upset someone else and not you. And there are generally only a few foods or food groups that you personally can't tolerate, but if you keep eating them, you'll damage the gut and become sensitive to more foods.

One of my clients, let's call her Sally, had Crohn's disease and was getting diarrhea constantly. Three, four times a day at least, she would have to run to the toilet. Obviously, this was very inconvenient for her life. Sally had quite a healthy diet. However, she had been on a low FODMAP diet for several years in the past.

FODMAP stands for Fermentable Oligosaccharides, Disaccharides, Monosaccharides and Polyols. They are a group of short-chain carbohydrates which are commonly poorly absorbed. The low FODMAP diet can help to relieve symptoms for IBS sufferers. The Monash University website has much more information on this.

As I mentioned earlier, a low FODMAP diet should be transitional in nature only and is not intended to be a long-term solution. It cuts out many beneficial fibres that create a healthy balance of gut bacteria.

We did some work to restore Sally's gut microbiome by feeding her gut bacteria healthy prebiotics and modifying her diet. We restored her gut garden. She's no longer got any urgent need to go to the bathroom and is only going twice per day as normal.

Restrictive diets aren't my preference. I find that the combination of fixing the system (see previous chapter) and some minor diet modifications or IGG food intolerance testing works best.

But the first step is to become aware of what you're eating now.

I always get my clients to record a diet and symptom diary. My client, Sally, really took to it and she continued to keep it for weeks afterwards.

She said that it really brought awareness to what she was eating, and it kept her on track because she had to record it all. She said that she could see certain things creeping in too often, and it also helped her to monitor how her symptoms improved as we continued our work together. This alone changed the way she viewed food and inspired her to eat better and to keep going.

There's a lot going on in your diet and with your symptoms that you simply won't realise. Studies indicate that your memory fades after 10 minutes and is replaced by perceptions. This means that you're not necessarily going to remember all your symptoms and what you ate.

You've also got a lot on your mind and your diet and symptoms will not be at the forefront. They may be to some extent, but you won't have the full awareness until you see it written out in front of you.

The point is, a diet and symptom diary is the perfect method for you to become self-aware of exactly what you're eating, and how you're feeling.

I've used it myself and it can be a little confronting.

Sometimes, when you look back at the week and you see the amount of 'one offs' and all the extra things that crept in, you can see how much it adds up. And you really see how often you're getting symptoms. You might know that they happen a lot but when you see written down it does make a difference.

The other point to be aware of is that food reactions can be delayed up to 72 hours. This means that you might eat something and not get symptoms for two days. But there's no way to remember this unless you see it written down, or have the proper testing done.

The food diary is so simple, yet so effective!

At this stage, we're gathering clues. We've got to first get a really good grip on what's happening right now in this moment. This is where you start. When you understand what's happening, what's actually in your diet and the symptoms that are actually happening, you're able to then look at this and identify patterns.

Once you've completed the diary, you can go back through and start highlighting some common themes. Maybe you notice that you eat a lot of dairy and you're also getting diarrhoea. Maybe you noticed that you were anxious one day and you had eaten fast food the day before. Perhaps you were bloated each day, and then you can have a look and see what you're eating consistently.

The other thing to look at is how often you're eating the more inflammatory foods. How often are you eating high processed, high sugar foods, takeaway, sugary snacks, coffee, alcohol? There's no judgement here. It's simply something to become aware of.

Of course, if you started eating more kindly for your body as I described in the previous chapter, hopefully your symptoms will have settled down a bit. This will help to narrow down the food.

Once you've highlighted some common patterns and you've gathered awareness of what's happening right now, we can start to heal your gut through using the power of food as medicine, which I'll explain in the next chapter.

For a step-by-step guide to this process, you'll find a link to download my free Ultimate Guide to Alleviating Gut Grief at the back of this book.

Activity

- Download my free Ultimate Guide to Alleviating Gut Grief (link at the back of the book) and complete it

- Keep a Diet & Symptom diary for 7 days (available in the download)

- Become aware of the correlations between your energy, mood, bowels and food

- Make changes as appropriate

Chapter 7 – Your Gut is You

"The art of healing comes from nature, not from the physician. Therefore, the physician must start from nature, with an open mind" – Paracelsus

At the end of the day your gut is you.

This is the biggest discovery I found in my health journey.

As part of my studies, and as part of my dedication to live a healthy life, I have eaten a mostly healthy and very strict gluten free diet ever since my diagnosis of coeliac disease.

I love eating healthy food. I love the way it makes my body feel. And I love creating new healthy recipes. I also love taking supplements. Sometimes maybe a little too much.

But the interesting thing that I found in my journey was that despite being on this great diet, taking all the right supplements and doing all the right things, my symptoms suddenly started coming back.

I was in pain all the time and had headaches constantly. I was exhausted again, and my gut started being all over the place with diarrhea some weeks constipation the next. I was getting reflux again. I just couldn't understand what was going on, and I was feeling worse and worse.

While I was studying, I did learn about the connection between the gut and the brain. But I didn't realise that it applied to me until I read *Rushing Women's Syndrome* by Dr Libby Weaver. There was something about her explanation of what constitutes a 'rushing woman' that finally made me see that I was in that space.

I had some emotional issues that I was ignoring, but more importantly, I finally understood that my stress was 95% internal. I knew that I was stressed, but I thought it was because of everything happening around me. Dr Libby's book made me realise that my stress was actually coming from within. This was the incredibly crucial piece that I was missing.

Once I addressed this and started to heal emotionally, my gut symptoms finally improved. And not only that but the confusion disappeared. I felt more confident in myself and more peaceful.

I'm sure you've felt your gut reacting to stress before. Whether that's a sinking feeling in the stomach, butterflies, a sharp sensation or even loose bowels when you're feeling nervous. And perhaps you notice that your symptoms get worse when you feel stressed, anxious, or depressed (which becomes a vicious cycle because your symptoms are also very stressful!).

There is more research coming out on the gut-brain connection almost every day, however, the concept is not a new one. The first official probiotic treatment for depression was implemented back in 1910[7].

This connection, called the gut-brain axis, operates via a two-way communication system. The gut has its own nervous system, the enteric nervous system, and it communicates with the brain via the vagus nerve which we discussed earlier in this book.

Remember, the body doesn't know what the thought is – only how the thought makes it feel. Thoughts and feelings of worry, anxiety, stress, depression, or anger all translate to the same thing according to the brain – danger. It prepares the body accordingly to get you out of danger by activating the sympathetic nervous system (SNS) or the 'flight or fight' response.

As mentioned earlier, the SNS essentially shuts down digestion by drawing blood away from your digestive tract and halting the secretion of digestive enzymes. If your life is in danger there is no need to waste energy on digestion!

The result is that you're not able to digest and absorb your food properly. Food particles ferment in the colon instead which causes gut symptoms even if you have your diet right. A food intolerance literally means 'an inability to digest a food'. If you're not digesting anything, you're going to be intolerant to everything.

In the previous chapters I've spoken about getting the balance of bacteria right in the gut, and this will help improve your mood. But we've also got to look after the brain, because your thought patterns and beliefs not only shape your health, they also shape how you approach your health.

You can have all the right information and be given the right tools and techniques, but whether you do it or not is largely going to depend on how you feel about yourself and your own level of self-worth. If you won't do self-care because you believe you don't deserve it or you believe there isn't time, and you never look after yourself, your health will continue to suffer.

The 'no time' factor is a big one. We're all more time poor than ever, we all have more pressures and demands to keep up with, and it feels like the Earth is spinning more quickly by the day. Whenever you ask someone how they are, the answer is usually 'busy'. But what does this kind of thinking do for our health, our ability to feel and experience life?

We need to explore this and dive into what *really* makes us feel like we have no time. And reframe the way we view self-care. Because self-care not selfish. In fact, it's our responsibility to look after ourselves so that we can be there for those we care about, and so that we don't inflict our pain on them.

We've got to let go the idea that you always must keep going and be on the go, because it's simply not helpful. No one can be on the go all the time. Our bodies weren't made for it and we weren't made for it.

The body literally breathes a sigh of relief when we give ourselves that permission to relax and let go, even just a little. When we drop our ideas of how things should be, how we should be, and when we start to relax into the flow of life gently and gradually. This is covered in more depth in later chapters.

You can't change external circumstances very often. The only thing you can change is how you talk to yourself, how you feel about yourself, the way you carry yourself and, in turn, the way you respond to those external situations.

One of my clients, Lynne, was feeling a little overwhelmed when I was talking about self-care. But when she saw that we weren't taking anything away and that she wasn't compromising on her capabilities or worth by incorporating a little bit of relaxation, she felt that she could give herself a break.

Lynne started by sitting in her chair for an extra 10 minutes after her ileostomy bag was changed, to give herself a chance to rest. And that was enough to start. That alone gave her some breathing room, helping her to calm her nervous system and reduce her gut symptoms.

Importantly, we also deepened into her beliefs around why she wasn't 'allowed' to relax in the first place.

Too many women I've worked have had such low self worth (myself included). But the thing is, if you weren't worthy, you wouldn't even be here. Because everything on this planet and even in our solar system exists for a purpose. Planet Earth gives us everything we need to thrive. Flowers have the sun and the rain. It's all connected and you're a part of this.

Please remember that you're worth looking after, that you're special, you matter and the people who love you just want you to be happy. When you approach your health from this space and this energy, it makes all the difference to how you heal.

Activity

- Write down at least 10 things you like about yourself. If you find this difficult, think harder.

- Then at the end write 'thank you more please'.

- Think about these things every time you look in the mirror.

Chapter 8 – Taming Tension

"If you're depressed, you're living in the past, if you're anxious you're living in the future, if you're at peace you're living in the present" – Buddha

Have you ever noticed how tense you are?

Or maybe you don't even realise it, because you're so used to it?

But you'll know about it if you ever get a massage because it hurts so much with all that tension you're carrying.

Perhaps even right now, your fists are clenched, your jaw is clenched, and perhaps you're even trying to rush through this book so that you can get onto the next thing. If this is you, pause and take a deep belly breath right now!

I recently saw a video of myself where I was skipping along, but what hit me was how rigid I was. I was surprised I didn't snap in half my body was so tight.

Anxiety has always been a big part of my life. I've always felt the pressure to perform well, be a good person, fit in, do a good job, keep everyone happy and create the perfect environment.

I was never very good at going with the flow and allowing instead of forcing. I refused to ride the wave and instead tried to control where it landed (spoiler alert: it didn't work).

Breaking this pattern was one of the most important things I've done. It took a lot of learning to trust, building of self-acceptance and, most importantly, processing my emotions instead of allowing them to store and fester inside me.

A client of mine, we'll call her Lisa, was putting a lot of pressure on herself (like so many of us do). She felt like she had to do everything herself and couldn't ask for help because she was at home all the time and didn't want to bother her partner. She had a lovely partner who was always happy to help, but she didn't want him to have to. As a result, she was carrying a lot of stress inside which was driving her gut symptoms.

She's now learned to accept help, release stored emotions, and be kinder to herself. Her symptoms settled and she's now feeling amazing.

Feelings of anxiety, stress, depression, or anger create a lot of tension in the body, especially if they are repressed. This tension drives the sympathetic nervous system (SNS) response which prevents you from absorbing your food. The SNS also impairs the body's ability to heal because it also stops your immune system from producing immune cells and it perpetuates inflammation in the body. It keeps you unhealthy and stuck.

Tension makes your body feel unsafe, which activates the SNS response in the body, and this essentially takes away any chance your body has of healing itself.

As your body fills up with emotions, it's a bit like a dam getting fuller and heavier. The pipes start behaving inefficiently, the sides start to crack, until it all becomes too much, and the dam breaks.

Emotions change the physiology of the body. Unprocessed emotions become stored in organs, muscle, skin, tissues and glands. These organs all have receptors on them which access and store emotional information. This means that emotional memory becomes stored in many places in the body, not just the brain.

This is why it's so important to have a practice in place to release this tension every day. Internal head talk is a big part of this, but there are other practices that you can put in place also.

Meditation is a very ancient, long-standing practice that, when practiced daily, has been proven to dampen genes involved in inflammation, create more neuroplasticity in the brain, improve memory, concentration, mental stamina and decrease depression and anxiety.

Importantly, meditation activates the parasympathetic nervous system (PNS) – also known as the 'rest and digest' state. This, as the name suggests, is ideal to support a healthy gut and digestive system.

The PNS is the state that humans are designed to spend most of the time in. It allows for proper digestion and absorption of food, a healthy immune system, balanced hormones and feelings of relaxation and peace.

Unfortunately, we now spend most of the time in sympathetic nervous system (SNS) dominance – the 'flight or fight' state. As I've mentioned earlier in the book, this is a major driver of the increase in digestive disorders that we are seeing today.

Alongside meditation, there are many other ancient practices such as tai chi and qigong which have the same effect on the body. I like qigong because it's a moving meditation and this can be nice to do when your brain is too hyperactive to sit down and meditate. To learn more about qigong, I recommend reading the work of Dr Nicholas Blewett at qifit.com.au.

The good news about meditation is that it doesn't have to be a proper sit-down practice for you to get the benefits. Simply bringing yourself into the present moment – feeling the clothes on your skin, noticing the food as you eat it, looking up at the sky – is a meditative practice and gives you similar benefits.

Another great way to relieve some of the tension and help your body relax is by moving emotions through the body. Bodywork such as massage, acupuncture or reiki can be great for this, but a daily practice of stretching, meditating, journaling or simply doing something you enjoy like a walk-in nature is helpful as well.

Activity

I'd like to share with you a technique based on a couple of teachings that I've learnt. I've incorporated some of my learnings from Gustavo Cestari from AMAR Centre for Mindfulness & Human Thriving, and I've infused it with a technique called circular breathing.

Gustavo taught me a lot about the practice of mindfulness. Importantly, I learned that you should never try to push down and bury your feelings.

Often when we get a bad or negative feeling the instinct is to push it away, get rid of it and ignore it. But this only creates more tension and encourages you to ignore your feelings rather than process them.

It's crucial to process your emotions, otherwise they come out through your digestion and detoxification organs – liver and kidneys – and cause symptoms.

Mindfulness is about bringing yourself back into the present and recognising that right now in this moment, you are safe. At the end of the day, your brain ultimately wants to know that you are safe, and it will only know that you are safe if you feel safe.

This is an activity you can do when you're feeling overwhelmed to help bring you back into balance.

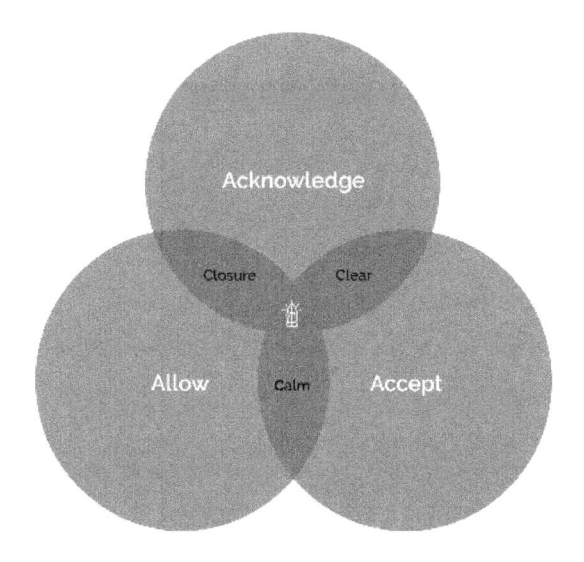

Essentially, you acknowledge the feelings that are there and accept them. Then you process them and allow them to move through the body. This helps to restore calm, clarity and gain closure on the situation.

Here are the steps:

1) Listen to the sounds you can hear in the room, outside the room, be aware of what is happening right at this moment.

2) Notice how you feel. Instead of trying to get rid of it or judging yourself for feeling that way, notice where in the body the sensation is. For example, if you feel anxious, do you feel it in your chest? Heart? Notice where in the body the emotion is sitting.

3) Scan the body for a pleasurable sensation or think about a time when you were grateful for something (the technique you choose here will depend on you). Where is the pleasurable sensation in the body? Is it the comfy chair, or maybe your clothes? Where is gratitude in the body?

4) Breathe and allow the sensations to mix together – let them integrate.

5) Open your eyes and notice how you feel.

Chapter 9 – Supercharge Your Self Love

"Loving ourselves works miracles in our lives" – Louise Hay

How do you feel when you read the words 'self-love'?

Does it make you feel uncomfortable, egotistical or is it even a foreign concept?

When I first mentioned the concept of self-love to my client Lynne, she had no idea how to respond. Because she had never even thought of it. She couldn't understand the idea of it.

So, we started with gratitude. Even if you're not where you want to be, you got yourself to where you are today, and that is always something to be grateful to yourself for.

I'm very happy to share with you that since Lynne and I did some more work around this, she feels much calmer and more able to tolerate abrupt changes. She's much more grounded, psychologically stable and stressful events don't set her gut off like they used to. She doesn't even need to take medication that she was taking before.

Self-love is a bit like a bank account. If you only take from it and never top it back up, it will slowly dwindle until there's nothing left. Then it takes even more work to get the levels back up to where they were.

We were born with a bank account filled with self-love. We didn't have the shame, guilt or embarrassment that comes as we get older. But without any maintenance during the negative experiences that happen during life, for many people this self-love disappears and is replaced by harsh self-talk and self-criticism. Criticism for all the things you say wrong, the mistakes you make and the people you upset. At least, from your perspective.

Many of us have ridiculously high standards for ourselves and if we don't meet these impossible standards every second of every day, we beat ourselves up for it. As my husband used to say to me 'you wouldn't even speak to a stranger on the street like that, so why you?'.

If you don't love yourself, you'll likely:

- Not believe compliments

- Brush off achievements as luck

- Not engage in self-care because of a belief that you don't deserve it

- Identify as being a perfectionist

- Not stand up for yourself

Research has uncovered that kind self-talk activates the relaxation response in the body – the 'rest and digest' response – the parasympathetic nervous system (PNS). As the name suggests, this is the state you want to be in for good digestion. On top of this, it has also been identified that negative self-talk activates the sympathetic nervous system (SNS).

When we spend too much time in the SNS, we are essentially in survival mode. Our bodies were not made to be in this state long-term. We were designed to be in the 'rest and digest' state 90% of the time (unless we were in physical danger).

Not only does the SNS shut down digestion, but it also messes with reproductive hormones, the immune system and the brain. And we spend most of our time in this state now, especially given the way we think and feel about ourselves. This must change, but the only way to truly change it is to change how you feel about yourself. To change the way you speak to yourself.

Watching internal language is so important. Even if you're doing some self care and eating well, but you're still talking to yourself negatively and putting yourself down, you'll stay in SNS dominance.

You may even only be doing self-care because it's something you think you *should* do, not something you feel like you *deserve*. There's a totally different energy in that. So, it's important to recognize how you speak to yourself and the way you think about yourself, so that you can reprogram this.

Rekindling self-love was a big part of my healing journey and to be honest, it's an ongoing process. I did go through some deep work a few years ago and was feeling quite good about things. As part of this, I set up some maintenance things for myself.

But then when life got a bit crazy with some huge changes, I didn't maintain these things. And before I knew it, all the negative self-talk, anxiety and frustration came back. My bloating was terrible, my reflux came back, and I was exhausted. I wasn't looking after myself at all.

Here's how to pull yourself out of self-criticism.

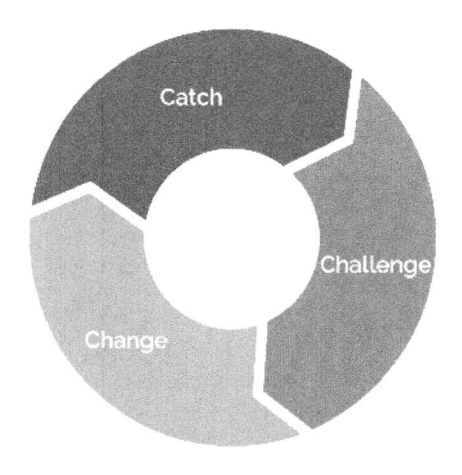

Start to catch your self-talk. Most of that you say to yourself happens unconsciously, so start by bringing it to the forefront of your mind. Notice the way you speak to yourself, where your thoughts go, and what you think when you look in the mirror. What do you say to yourself with something goes wrong, or you make a mistake, or you aren't 'perfect'?

Is it compassionate or judgmental and harsh? Is it something you'd say to your friends, family or even someone on the street?

This is where we challenge the thought. For example, if you drop something, and you automatically think 'I can't do anything right', challenge that. If you can't do anything right, you wouldn't be here today. It's impossible to live and not do anything right. So, it's an untrue thought.

Bring some curiosity to this situation too – what put this thought there and why did your mind automatically turn to criticism?

Then flip that criticism to encouragement.

When you look in the mirror, focus on the things that you like about yourself. Be grateful for all that your body gives you and does for you.

If you drop something, smile and pick it up, without the judgment. If anything, dropping things are a sign to be gentle with yourself and give yourself some rest. Get curious about the situation instead of being so quick to judge yourself.

Let's now go a little deeper.

Often, when we have this negative self-talk going on constantly, there are things we haven't forgiven ourselves for. Things that we feel ashamed of or are still beating ourselves up for, or situations where we haven't lived up to our own impossible standards.

This was a big part of my personal healing journey as well. Every time I felt happy or proud, it was short-lived because suddenly an old memory would slap across my brain and I'd feel anxious and ashamed. I felt like I didn't deserve to be happy or have achievements, because of something I said or did years ago. I couldn't accept compliments and I'd never feel proud of myself.

It took some digging over a period of a couple of years to really move past this. Logically I knew it was silly, but logical doesn't always prevail in the face of emotions!

Eventually, I was able to look at my past through the lenses of an outsider and I could see that everything I ever said or did, everything I was ashamed of, I only did it because I wanted to be loved and accepted. I would compromise on myself to try and 'fit in'. But once I really understood this, from a place of compassion, it was like a huge weight had literally been lifted from my shoulders and I could breathe again. And my body said, 'thank you'.

Any relationship requires respect. If two people don't respect each other, care for each other and look after each other, the health of the relationship will deteriorate. It's the same as your relationship with yourself.

There may be something (or many things) you haven't forgiven yourself for or things that you still cringe over and feel embarrassed about. Past experiences you haven't let go of.

If this is you, remember that hindsight is 20/20 vision. It's all too easy to look back and think of what you 'should' or 'shouldn't' have done. But at the end of the day, we all do our best with the information we had and the emotional resources available to us at that point in time.

So, forgive yourself. We're human, which means we make mistakes. It's what we do! We forgive others for their mistakes all the time – so why is it any different for you?

This is so important to do because if you continually look back on these situations and judge yourself for things in the past, it will hold your health back for the rest of your life.

Once you heal your relationship with yourself, you start looking after yourself better. You feed yourself better, prioritise yourself and feel better about yourself. You give your body what it needs to heal and spend more time in the parasympathetic nervous system (PNS) state which allows your body to activate its natural healing mechanisms. You become more intuitive, start to recognise what's best for you, and you respect your body. All of this helps your gut to heal.

Activity

Write yourself a love letter. Look at yourself from an outsider's perspective. Write the letter as though you're writing it to a close friend. Congratulate them on all they've achieved. Show them compassion for all the tough times they've been through and encourage them for making it through the other side. Tell them to look after themselves. Write down all the people who care about them and who they care about. Give yourself the same care that you would give another.

Read this letter whenever you're going through a tough time or feeling down on yourself.

Also, write down 10 things you're proud of yourself for that happened within the last week. Perhaps it's meeting a deadline, preparing a delicious dinner, or making it through a recent challenge. The point of this is to teach yourself to focus on the things you're proud of yourself for, instead of only focusing on the negative.

This activity helps to train your brain to think that way, and it also helps you to feel motivated and better about yourself.

Make this list every week. Eventually, your internal language will follow. And each time something negative does come up, you catch it, you challenge it, and you change it. You get to decide what goes on in your head – no one else.

Chapter 10 – Sustainable Solutions

"You can't afford to get sick, and you can't depend on the present health care system to keep you well. It's up to you to protect and maintain your body's innate capacity for health and healing by making the right choices in how you live" – Andrew Weil

Often when self-care is suggested, or when I suggest for self-care to my clients, I get some resistance. They look at me like 'that sounds nice, but I don't have time for that! When am I going to find time – I don't even have time to breathe and you want me to spend 10 minutes per day meditating??'

Or they tell me that they've tried to do some of these things, but their mind was too active, and it didn't work.

One of my clients struggled with the concept of taking time for herself because she believed that she was being lazy or ignoring her responsibilities. The idea of letting herself relax felt so foreign and unachievable. She couldn't sit still without thinking of all the other things she 'should' be doing.

Once she realised that the two can co-exist and made some minor changes to give herself some space, her pain and symptoms started to go down. She continued to grow this, and her gut no longer reacts to stressful events. She was surprised at how changing the way she thinks, even subtly, can be so powerful.

It's important that we all have our own self-care practices that we incorporate into every single day. We all need space to help us through difficult situations and even our daily lives.

We're all busy and there is a lot for our brains to worry about with so much bad news and negativity thrown at us every day. Research has shown that exposure to negative events, even events we are not directly involved in, can increase depressive symptoms in susceptible people.

When there's a lot going on self-care is usually the first thing to go. But that's when you need it the most because it's the thing that will help you to handle these stressful times.

Without our own space, we spend too much time in the sympathetic nervous system (SNS) dominance which causes us to become reactive and easily flustered. But, when we do take the time to calm our nervous system every single day, we become more resilient and are able to handle stressful situations with much more ease.

For example, if you've had a huge week, are feeling exhausted, and you get home and see that the dishwasher hasn't been unstacked when you asked for it to be done, you're more likely to snap. But if you've had a huge week *and* you've supported yourself during it, that same situation is less likely to bother you.

Most importantly, by spending as much time as possible in parasympathetic nervous system (PNS) dominance, you're enabling the natural healing mechanisms of the body to switch on. Your food is being digested properly and your gut remains calm.

Your Sustainable Solutions should be things you can commit to every single day. Things that you look forward to. And don't need to be big things. This shouldn't be a source of stress. It should be a rejuvenating activity that you like to do.

Breath-based work is the simplest way to calm your nervous system and reduce digestive symptoms. This is because deep belly breathing signals to the brain that you are safe. It's the quickest way to activate the relaxation response in the body, which is why it's so incredibly helpful for your digestion to take a few deep breaths before a meal.

Deep breathing takes you out of the past or future and brings you back to the present. This tells the brain that you are safe. If you can remind the brain that everything is okay every single day, it's going to go a long way to improving your digestion. In fact, you really need to be doing this in conjunction with any gut health plan, otherwise it simply won't work.

A great way to incorporate more calm into your life is to start the day off with a breath-based activity. This gives you that personal space we all need and sets the tone for your day ahead. Importantly, do something just for yourself before you check emails or social media.

For a long time, my morning routines were quite intense. I'd get up at the crack of dawn, have a pre-workout and go do a high intensity fitness class or gym session. Then I'd rush to work, have another coffee, and continue with my adrenaline fuelled day.

I did this because I thought I needed to exercise intensely all the time to look good. But I *never* believed that I looked good, so I continued to work out more and more. And my gut was constantly reminding me that I didn't feel good.

Ever since I started doing more yoga, meditation or qigong and stopped basing my exercise on high-intensity routines only, I've felt calmer, more mentally stable, and I don't think I look bad anymore! I also have more energy and am more productive when I start the day from a calm place.

Of course, there's nothing wrong with morning exercise. However, intense exercise does activate the SNS, so if you're already in SNS dominance, exercise like this is only going to wind you up even more.

It's also important to be aware of your head talk when you exercise. Do you do it to move your body and build strength, or is it something you feel like you have to do to lose weight and you therefore go as hard as possible while feeling bad about the way you look? Do you do yoga to celebrate your body or are you more focused on being able to do the advanced poses?

I still go to the gym but I'm no longer obsessed with how I look which makes it much less stressful. I'm advancing my yoga practice but in a playful way, not an obsessive way.

Check in with how you're feeling about yourself when you exercise. And choose an exercise that you actually enjoy and which makes you feel good. It doesn't matter if you don't currently have an exercise schedule. All you really need to do is move your body daily. Perhaps you could get up 15 minutes earlier and do some gentle yoga or go for a walk.

Another nice way to start your day is by pulling back the curtains and taking in the morning sun. This gives you a natural boost of serotonin to brighten your mood for the day.

Remember, the purpose of all of this is to calm your nervous system and reduce your digestive symptoms. I can't stress enough how much this matters.

Activity

Choose a self-care practice that you can commit to twice per day.

Here's a list of suggestions to get you started:

- 10 deep belly breaths on waking
- 10 minutes guided meditation
- 20 minutes yoga or stretching sequence
- Attend a restorative yoga / qigong / tai chi class
- Attend a gym class like Body Balance
- Go for a 30 minute walk
- Drink 2L water
- Before bed, write down 5 good things that happened that day
- 15 minutes gentle stretching before bed
- Dim the lights and avoid technology 1 hour before bed
- Leave all technology outside of the bedroom
- Read a book
- Listen to music

- Catch up with a friend

Don't worry about starting small because the little things add up.

One client started with a 5-minute guided breathing meditations twice per day using her Apple watch. She would do one whilst waiting for a coffee, and the other just before bed. This gave her the breathing room that she needed without having her time taken away from anything else.

Chapter 11 – Harmonious Healing

"Gratitude for the present moment and the fullness of life now is the true prosperity" – Eckhart Tolle

I read a story recently which had a big impact on me.

In this story, there were three beggars. Each beggar was given a bowl of food. The first beggar was given a full bowl of food, but the next two were only given half a bowl. The second beggar felt resentful because he only got half and ate his feeling resentful. However, the third beggar ate his meal with gratitude for what he had been given.

These two people reacted entirely differently to the exact same situation (and you can imagine who actually absorbed the nutrients from that meal). In other words, they both decided how they would respond.

You have this same choice every day. You can choose to see all that is lacking, or you can choose to be grateful for everything that you do have.

You might be wondering how you can feel grateful when you've got these gut symptoms that are ruining everything you try to do.

One way to release the hold that your symptoms have on you is to look at what they have given you.

When I was diagnosed with coeliac disease, I was very resentful of all the things I couldn't eat. I hated having to find gluten free places, ask questions about the menu and get the eye rolls (coeliac disease wasn't as well understood then), and I was very upset when I discovered what gluten free bread was like (this has also come a long way!).

But in reality, my diagnosis gave me my health back. Coeliac disease was what finally kicked me into gear and got me to eat healthily, exercise more and look after myself better. Coeliac disease was what inspired me to study nutritional medicine. It led me down this path where I've met so many people, done so much healing and have been lucky enough to help many other people manage their gut issues too.

What has your digestive disorder given you?

When you don't have gratitude, you can never feel satisfied. It's not possible to feel fulfilled or see all the good in your life. This can make you feel a lot of resentment, distrust, and even anxiety. All of which disrupts your nervous system, drives the production of cortisol and adrenaline, and upsets your gut. Practicing gratitude changes your biochemistry, improves your quality of life, and helps your gut heal.

Gratitude is one of the most studied emotions in human history.

Research by The Happy Human demonstrated that gratitude journaling increases longevity by 10%. It helps you to live 10% longer.

Research by Positive Psychology Process found that keeping a gratitude journal decreases depressive symptoms by 30%, and research from The Grateful Heart revealed that feelings of gratitude activates the parasympathetic nervous system (PNS). This means that it switches off the sympathetic nervous system (SNS) and allows the body to enter a state of healthy digestion and healing.

Gratitude distracts your brain from being stressed because the brain can only focus on one thing at a time. You feel less stressed when you're more focused on being grateful.

This doesn't mean that you should ignore stress and anxiety. Negative emotions still need to be processed as I described in chapter 8. However, a very effective way to stop your gut reacting to everything, and to feel healthier and happier, is have a daily gratitude practice.

Practice training your brain to become aware of things that you're grateful for. And don't place a judgment on it and think that what you feel grateful for isn't 'good enough'. Good enough only exists in your head, nowhere else.

Avoid the temptation to feel guilty that you have all these wonderful things that you don't appreciate right now. This doesn't help your nervous system to feel any better. Forgive yourself and move on. The more you focus on appreciation, the more you will feel it.

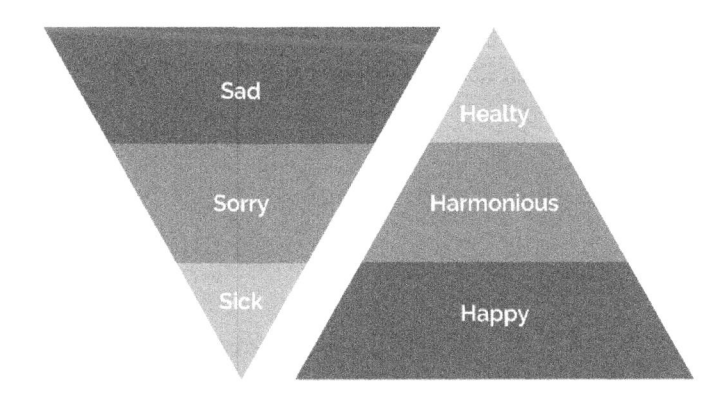

[Diagram: Two triangles. Left inverted triangle labeled top to bottom: Sad, Sorry, Sick. Right upright triangle labeled top to bottom: Healty, Harmonious, Happy.]

When you spend most of your time feeling sad and sorry for yourself, it makes you sick. But when you spend your time feeling happy and in harmony, this helps you to be healthy both physically and emotionally.

The reason we all need a daily gratitude practice is because we aren't conditioned to feel grateful. We live in a world where we are faced with so much negativity. There's so much fear about time, money, death, war, disease and all the things that can go wrong. We're so connected now which is great, but it also means we're exposed to all the bad things happening in the world all the time. This can keep you in SNS dominance if you don't give yourself a break.

is also designed to find the fear because the brain's job is to keep us alive. It finds the danger and tells you to stay away from it. This strategy has kept us alive for a very long time. But we are no longer facing the same dangers that we used to. So, we forget to enjoy the moment, and we forget that there's so much to be grateful for every single day.

If you don't notice the good in your life now, you never will. It's easy to fall into the trap of thinking that you'll be happy when you have no symptoms, more money, a different job, bigger house, able to travel more or whatever it is. But it's an illusion because even when you get the thing, you end up feeling the same.

There was a period in my life when I moved 11 times in 5 years. I kept thinking that when I got to the next place / lived with these people / changed cities / lived overseas I would be happy. It didn't work.

What I wouldn't understand until years later is that the situation isn't what makes us unhappy. Our beliefs about the situation, or our beliefs about why we have to stay in that situation, are what make us unhappy.

It's awful when we do lose something or someone, and we wish we had appreciated what we had before. The present moment is all we have.

Whenever I'm feeling overwhelmed or bogged down, I like to put it all into perspective. I remember that we are spinning on a rock in an infinite Universe and there is so much more to life than what I can see in that moment. I think about what this situation is here to teach me.

If you're having trouble feeling grateful, get into nature. Look around at all the different colours, trees, animals, waterfalls, flowers, mountains, and oceans. Appreciate the way nature operates and supports itself, and therefore supports you. Our planet gives us everything we need. Be grateful that you get to witness and experience all of this.

We are all here on this planet and we've built roads, plumbing, sewerage systems and electricity so we can enjoy travel, fresh water, food and all the comforts that we have.

Be grateful for your family, friends, job, home, and furniture. Even if it doesn't look or feel exactly the way you'd like, it's giving you what you need to stay alive. Be grateful for the fact that you can sleep safely in your bed at night.

This might sound silly, fluffy, or trivial, but if we don't appreciate what we've got, all too soon it will be gone. Life is moving faster and the only way to slow it down is to appreciate the present moment. The most effective way to stop feeling rushed, resentful, anxious, on edge, depressed or stressed is to bring gratitude in.

The best thing about this is that you'll start attracting more things that make you feel grateful. You give life to what you focus on. If you have two gardens and only water one, the other one will die. If all you focus on is what's going wrong, those thoughts will be all that occupies your mind.

The more you cultivate gratitude, the more natural and easier it becomes.

Activity

Each morning before you get out of bed, instead of stressing about what's ahead, take a deep breath and think about something you're looking forward to that day.

Are you looking forward to seeing your partner, your kids, your friends at work, your morning coffee? We need to train the brain to focus on these things, rather than the negative.

And start a gratitude journal.

Personally, I have a journal next to my bed and each night I write down at least five good things that happened that day. It forces me to see the good in each day and puts me into a positive frame of mind before going to sleep. It could be that I enjoyed the feeling of the warm sun, I received a nice compliment, or I enjoyed my nourishing breakfast. The important thing is not to judge what you write down.

This can be difficult on tough days when you've had a flare up or are in severe pain. But that's when it's even more important to cultivate gratitude, because it helps you to move through the more difficult times and pull yourself out of a negative spiral.

Remember, the present moment is all we have. If we aren't grateful, we become resentful and never see the good in life. Gratitude decreases pain, decreases gut symptoms, it activates the natural healing mechanisms in the body and increases longevity.

There's always, no matter what, something to be grateful for. Practice leaning into this and it will make all the difference to your symptoms.

Chapter 12 – Infusing Inspiration

"Live with intention. Walk to the edge. Listen hard. Practice wellness. Play with abandon. Laugh. Choose with no regret. Continue to learn. Appreciate your friends. Do what you love. Live as if this is all there is" – Mary Anne Radmacher

A common theme in my clients is that their issues started at a time in their lives when they were under huge amounts of pressure.

Some examples include the pressure of high school exams, of University, or being a new mum. We all feel pressure for different reasons, and our reasons will depend on the beliefs we have about ourselves and how we believe we need to perform or outwardly appear. But what we do have in common is that most of us do feel the pressure from somewhere.

One of my patterns is to work. And I mean *work*. I have always worked hard, to the point where nothing else matters. This was conditioning to some extent, working in stressful corporate environments for 10 years, but it was also something deeper. That environment only affected me in that way because of beliefs I had about myself.

I would neglect healthy eating, exercise, and my relationships to get the work done, the assignments in, and stay on top of the chores. I didn't even know that I was doing this until suddenly I realised how disconnected I was from everyone, even those closest to me. I suddenly saw that I never spoke to people or did anything just for fun. What even is 'fun'?

I thought the problem was my job and that my home business would fix it. But your patterns are your patterns, and I very quickly filled up all my time with work and nothing else. I wanted to do a good job and I didn't want to let anyone down. I was doing all the same things.

The thing with 'work' is that it's *never* done. Even if you worked 24/7 there would be more to do. It's common to think 'I'll get this task done, fix this task up and then I'll relax'. Then you rush through the tasks frantically, try to relax, but then remember all the *other* things you should be doing, and the guilt sets in.

Working constantly and never allowing yourself that time to rest and restore drives sympathetic nervous system (SNS) dominance. It increases cortisol and adrenaline, shuts down digestion and never gives your body a chance to heal. Neglecting your health in this way is a fast-track to a serious health crisis.

When did life get so serious and all about 'getting through it' as my husband loves to say. What happened to fun, connection, and happiness? Is this just a foreign concept that we just don't have time for anymore? Something we feel like we don't deserve?

Many of us spend too much time in the past or in the future. We're ruminating over past events and what we should have done/said differently, or we're worrying about future events which haven't happened yet (and may not ever happen).

This means that we miss the joy of the present moment. We don't notice the birds singing, the sun setting or the flowers blooming. Instead, our minds are preoccupied with work, negative head talk or other demands. Life becomes all about tasks instead of living, and before you know it the years fly by.

50% of happiness is based on your genetics, 10% on external circumstances and 40% comes from internal beliefs. This is why it's so important to align your internal beliefs with how you want to feel. Your own belief systems are the biggest factor in how you approach your health and your life.

We often believe that we have to live a certain way, have certain things, be this or that, stay on top of everything and never fall behind. Because that's what many of us have been told and how we've been conditioned.

But the secret is you get to choose. You get to choose how you feel and you get to choose how you design your life. And the irony is that you *do* design your life without even realising it. You're always making decisions and adopting behaviours that create your life to be a certain way.

A close mentor of mine helped me to see this. She also said something that stuck with me, which was 'you've got to make time for the things you do want, or you'll get what you don't want'. Food for thought.

Most of us never even think about what we really want. And if we do, we often think that what we want is irresponsible, impossible, or perhaps we even feel that we don't deserve it. We all have dreams and desires burning inside our soul. We all have things that we want in life. And yet we very rarely give ourselves permission to go for it.

Healing your gut and living your life with little to no symptoms is absolutely, 100% possible for you. Even if you feel more confused than ever. I wholeheartedly believe in you.

You don't need to have the whole journey mapped out. You don't need to know how it will happen (chances are, it'll happen in a way you could never have imagined). All you need to do is act on the urges leading you along the path. Act on your intuition.

You weren't born to live in pain, to have your health go from bad to worse, to feel anxious and confused on a daily basis, to worry about what food is doing to your body or to feel like there's no hope for anything better.

You are allowed to enjoy nourishing meals, to have a fulfilling social life with strong relationships, to progress your passions, to see the world, and have all the experiences that you want from life.

It's time to set the intention to heal your gut, the way you would set an intention to achieve any goal in your life.

For example, if your goal was to get a promotion at work, perhaps you would study the new role, put in extra hours and compile a list of reasons of why you are the right person for that position.

Maybe you would get excited about it and bring that passion and enthusiasm to your work every day. You might openly share how committed you are to the company and how much more you could bring to the table.

If you took the opposite attitude and figured you would never get the promotion so why even bother, what do you think your chances are?

In the words of Henry Ford, "Whether you think you can, or you think you can't – you're right".

You cannot heal your gut with diet and supplements alone. But if you also do the mindset work, and you let yourself believe that you can recover from your health issues, there really is no stopping you.

Activity

A very effective way to reach your goal is to imagine how it feels to have it right now.

If you want to have less gas, for example, but thinking about it makes you anxious because you don't think it's possible, your brain isn't going to be motivated to achieve that goal. But if you imagine how good it will feel once you do have less gas, how much easier life will be, and how much less embarrassed you are, this generates emotions of hope and motivation, which help you to keep going. When you're in this frame of mind you notice opportunities and act more quickly and, therefore, you get the health you want much faster.

Write down your top gut health goals and the things you'd like to do once you have fewer symptoms.

Do you want less bloating, gas and gut pain? Would you like regular bowels so that you don't have to feel anxious and awkward about being in public places? Do you want more energy, to return to work, to travel, to see your family more and reconnect with friends?

Notice the thoughts and feelings that come up as you write these down. If you feel nervous, explore that. Are you nervous that you won't be able to do it? Do you feel angry because it hasn't happened yet?

Remember, no judgment. This is about awareness.

Then change the language to present tense. If you wrote 'I want less gas after eating' change it to 'I have less gas after eating'. Notice how this feels in the body.

Tell yourself this every single day. Give yourself permission to embrace the relief, excitement, and gratitude that you feel. Get specific and imagine how it will feel to eat lunch and head back to your desk without any discomfort.

In the famous words usually attributed to Walt Disney, "if you can dream it, you can do it".

End Note

I hope that this book has helped you to understand the fundamentals of gut healing and how you can restore your own gut garden with a nourishing diet, a clean environment, and a healthy mindset.

We've covered:

- Why being diagnosed with a digestive disorder doesn't mean your life is over

- How to listen to your body and get your diet right for you

- The gut-brain connection and what this means for gut health

- The impact that your internal beliefs and thought patterns have on your gut symptoms

- Techniques to process and release negative emotions so they don't come out in your digestion

- Reframing negative feelings about your health

- Brain hacks to help you achieve your gut health goals quickly

At the end of the day, this is what health all about. It's not just about the physical symptoms that you're experiencing. It's also about how you feel about yourself and about life.

It's very easy to prioritise everything else above our health. But the truth is, we can't do any of those things without our health.

One of my mentors says that if you lose a car, you can buy another one. But if you lose your health, you'll spend the rest of your life trying to get it back. He's spot on.

So, it's time to take care of yourself and your gut. And start *right now*.

Whatever you're feeling inspired to do in this moment, go do it! Acting on your inspired ideas is the secret to getting your health back as quickly as possible.

Keep going, keep believing, be patient and never give up.

References

[1] Gastroenterological Society of Australia, 2018. Irritable Bowel Syndrome. Retrieved from https://www.gesa.org.au/resources/patients/irritable-bowel-syndrome/

[2] Canavan, C., West, J., & Card, T. (2014). The epidemiology of irritable bowel syndrome. Clinical epidemiology, 6, 71–80. https://doi.org/10.2147/CLEP.S40245

[3] GBD 2017 Inflammatory Bowel Disease Collaborators. (2017). The global, regional, and national burden of inflammatory bowel disease in 195 countries and territories, 1990–2017: a systematic analysis for the Global Burden of Disease Study 2017. The Lancet Gastroenterology & Hepatology, 5(1), 17-30. doi: https://doi.org/10.1016/S2468-1253(19)30333-4

[4] Crohn's & Colitis Australia & PricewaterhouseCoopers Australia. (2013). Improving Inflammatory Bowel Disease Care Across Australia. Retrieved from https://www.crohnsandcolitis.com.au/site/wp-content/uploads/PwC-Report-2013-Executive-Summary.pdf

[5] Crohn's & Colitis Foundation of America. (2014). The Facts About Inflammatory Bowel Disease. Retrieved from https://www.crohnscolitisfoundation.org/sites/default/files/2019-02/Updated%20IBD%20Factbook.pdf

[6] Blaser, M. J., & Falkow, S. (2009). What are the consequences of the disappearing human microbiota?. Nature reviews. Microbiology, 7(12), 887–894. https://doi.org/10.1038/nrmicro2245

[7] Evrensel, A., & Ceylan, M. E. (2015). The Gut-Brain Axis: The Missing Link in Depression. Clinical psychopharmacology and neuroscience : the official scientific journal of the Korean College of Neuropsychopharmacology, 13(3), 239–244. https://doi.org/10.9758/cpn.2015.13.3.239

About The Author

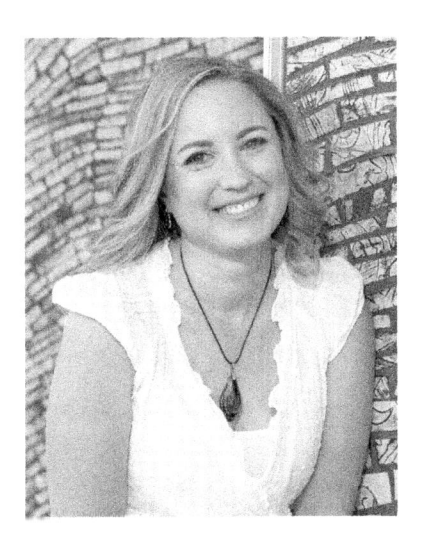

Sarah Spann

Sarah brings passion, understanding, personal insight and professional expertise to help people to heal their gut, relieve their symptoms and get back to feeling like the healthiest, most vibrant versions of themselves.

As a highly sought-after nutritionist and coach, Sarah has a unique ability to put all the pieces of the digestive puzzle together to facilitate quick and long-lasting results.

Based on her own experiences, Sarah has a special interest in helping people recover from digestive disorders including irritable bowel syndrome, inflammatory bowel disease and coeliac disease.

She believes that healing the gut not only requires the right awareness and understanding of the way the gut works, but that the mind must also be healed and strengthened to achieve optimum, long-term gut health.

"I began my journey around my mid-teenage years when I started to become quite unwell. I was underweight, often sick, my stomach was reacting to basically everything and I was constantly fatigued. Things continued to get worse as I got into my early twenties, and it was at the point where I was regularly going home from work and isolating myself because of it all. I was even hospitalised at one stage due to the pain, but no one ever knew what the problem was.

I was eventually diagnosed with coeliac disease in 2012. A few months later my symptoms were better, I had much more energy, I was at a healthy weight and my confidence was up.

But then things plateaued. Yes, I had improved, but I still had lots of gut symptoms, and my emotional state was all over the place.

Once I finally got to the bottom of what was really going on, I was able to address it and my health turned a corner for good.

When you have a digestive disorder your gut will always require maintenance, but knowing what your gut needs is what makes all the difference"

Sarah's unique understanding, through her own experience and her dedication to her many clients, has provided her with an insight that others don't have and this has led her to create and develop a holistic solution that addresses all factors which cause people to suffer from gut issues.

Sarah has completed a Bachelor of Health Science (Nutritional Medicine) and an Advanced Diploma of Nutritional Medicine. She is a registered practitioner with the Australian Traditional Medicine Society. Sarah's work has been featured in many publications including Healthline, The Good Seed Kefir Co., FodShopper, Australian Online Courses and Health Magazine UK.

To learn more about Sarah and her work, head to her website https://sarahspann.net.